ARTHRITIS

THE PAIN OF THE CENTURY

HOW TO PREVENT AND RELIEVE ARTHRITIS

MARK DUBE

Arthritis
Pain of the century
How to Prevent and Relieve Arthritis

ISBN-13: 978-1502413994
ISBN-10: 150241399X

Almost 1 in 2 people may develop knee arthritis by age of 85 years. Two among three obese persons may develop knee arthritis. A quarter of population experiences painful hip arthritis in their lifetime. According to current estimates, almost 52.5 million adults suffer from one or other form of arthritis in the United States. And by 2030, this number is projected to rise to 67 million. Arthritis can affect any joint of the body and cause debilitating effects on the patient. It neither kills nor allows an individual to live a healthy life.

This book introduces you to the science of arthritis and teaches you all the aspects of it to tackle your arthritis or prevent future occurrence. The book covers various aspects of arthritis:

- The meaning and types of arthritis
- The symptoms and treatment options for arthritis
- Home remedies and instant help tips
- And the wonders of cayenne pepper

CONTENTS

1. WHAT EXACTLY IS ARTHRITIS?

Arthritis is a disease that affects millions. This disease is one of those that get deep into the body causing one to avoid certain activities and life's pleasures. Though it is true that some people have used their Arthritis to useful means (such as predicting the weather because the Arthritis flares up), the disease is nothing that one would aspire to catch (It is one of the most painful experience the body should not go through).

Arthritis is inflammation in the joints. It is most associated with older people because their joints have had a lot more use than younger people have. Generally, the pain is found in the knees and the elbows. However, it has been known to occur in other areas of the body as well. Arthritis causes aches and pains in afflicted people. This is due to the bone rubbing against bone instead of being properly cushioned when movement is required. It can also cause joints stiffen, restricting mobility and making hands or feet of little or no use.

Arthritis was not brought to light until the year 1800 when a French medical student wrote a paper on the subject. Augustin-Jacob Landre-Beauvails wrote his doctoral thesis on a debilitating disease attacking the joints, but it was not until 1859 that the term Arthritis was used. It was called a new disease and was said that it would disappear by the end of the century. The reason the "New Disease" did not simply disappear was the suspected origin of the disease.

Archeologists have discovered evidence of arthritis in dinosaur fossils. This could possibly be the origin of the disease, but evidence points a different source, sugar. By 1771, sugar trade netted England 326,000 pounds annually. Sugar was still very expensive. Therefore, it was an indulgence only for the rich. In 1773 The Boston Tea Party took place bringing sugar prices down to a level where the middle class was able to afford it. From 1755 to 1765 sugar trading between Europe and the West Indies was at its peak. By 1800 England was trading 160 million pounds of sugar per year bringing in annual revenue of 3 million pounds. That is quite a bit of increase in sugar sales. This was the time when arthritis first appeared, according to Augustin-Jacob and then named in 1859. History further records that in 1874 Prime Minister Gladstone abolished the sugar tax. This made sugar cheaper, thus making it available to the masses. A steady increase in sugar consumption is the likely cause of the arthritis epidemic that is plaguing so many people today.

ARTHRITIS

2. INSTANT ARTHRITIS RELIEF IS POSSIBLE

Arthritis can be tricky to treat for the simple fact that it can be difficult to distinguish a simple muscle ache from an arthritis flare up. Instant arthritis relief is possible with topical creams and gels. There are a few main types of topical creams. Topical creams are typically used by patients whose body will not respond to oral treatments. It is highly recommended to consult a physician before starting a topical cream regime. These can be used every day for temporary relief from joint pain caused by arthritis.

The first of these topical relief agents is called counterirritants. These work to distract from the pain. Counterirritants cause the skin to feel either cold or hot. The cold or hot feeling essentially tricks the brain to make it focus on the irritation of the skin rather than the joint pain. Counterirritants use various oils and temperature variant substances to accomplish the goal of pain reduction. There are many substances in these counterirritants to accomplish pain relief.

- **Menthol** is a natural ingredient that offers both cooling and heating effects. Menthol has been used in Japan for over 2000 years, but was not adopted into western medicine until 1771. Menthol is derived from peppermint oil in its natural form. It is low in toxins, therefore has little irritation or side effects. Menthol is able to permeate deep into skin to temporarily relieve mild arthritis pain. The first sensation to the skin is that of a cool feeling as the menthol is penetrating the epidermis. This cooling sensation is followed by a warm feeling that relaxes the joints so that inflammation can be reduced.

- **Oil of Wintergreen** is often used in topical creams for its warming effects. The main ingredient in oil of wintergreen is methyl salicylate. Methyl salicylate is highly toxic and is a cousin to aspirin. Anyone allergic to aspirin is advised not to use any product containing oil of wintergreen. Symptoms of allergic reaction include redness, swelling, tightness or pain in chest, and swelling of lips, throat, or mouth. If these symptoms occur, seek immediate medical attention. Any persons on warfarin therapy should avoid the use of oil of wintergreen as it can react with the medicines for this therapy. It is also recommended that oil of wintergreen not be used on children, pregnant women, breastfeeding mothers, asthma patients, those with gastrointestinal inflammation, and persons with gastric irritation.

• **Camphor** is oil derived from the Camphor Laurel evergreen tree in Asia. Chinese traditionalists argue that for the most powerful camphor oil the tree must be at least 50 years old. This has not been proven by science but held in tradition by Chinese herbalists. Camphor is very powerful in raw form and should not be taken orally. Camphor is mostly found in balms or salves and has been mixed with other effective herbs to avoid toxicity. The FDA has approved concentrations of between 3 and 11% for over the counter use of camphor. Camphor is used in substances such as Vicks Vapor Rub to relieve minor aches and pains. Camphor numbs the nerve endings in skin so signals of pain cannot be sent to the brain, thus a temporary relief to arthritis pain.

• **Eucalyptus** is a type of tree. The oils and leaves of the Eucalyptus tree are what are used to make medicines. Eucalyptus in raw form must be diluted and applied to the skin for temporary relief of minor aches and pains. Eucalyptus should never be taken orally unless recommended by a doctor. Even taking Eucalyptus by mouth in small amounts can result in fatal circumstances. Eucalyptus is not to be applied to broken skin or used on children.

• **Turpentine oil** is only used in small doses in creams. Turpentine is derived from the long leaf pine tree. It causes a warming sensation to reduce pain and inflammation caused by arthritis. Turpentine is toxic if ingested. Even in small doses, turpentine can be fatal. Turpentine should not be used by pregnant or breastfeeding women and should never be given to children.

- **Dihydrochloride** works to relax muscles and reduce inflammation in joints. Dihydrochloride is sometimes referred to as histamine. Unlike other ingredients in many arthritis creams, dihydrochloride does not cause burning or irritation. It offers a fresh aroma that is pleasing rather than harsh, like with other creams. Dihydrochloride does not require a prescription and can be purchased anywhere arthritis creams are sold.

These ingredients are combined into a variety of creams and salves to offer much needed counterirritant pain relief. Some of these over the counter medications are Arthricare, Eucalyptamint, Icy Hot, and Therapeutic Mineral, Ice.

Another type of topical cream that is commonly used is known as salicylates. Unlike counterirritants, which distract from the pain at hand, salicylates have true pain relieving qualities. Much like aspirin is taken orally; these salicylates are the cream form of aspirin. They are applied directly into the skin and are absorbed at the source of the pain.When people hear the word "aspirin" they automatically think of the effects of oral aspirin which thin the blood. Salicylates, on the other hand, since they are applied to the skin and have a very low dose of aspirin, are unlikely to cause thinning of the blood, so they are safe in that regard. There are a number of salicylates on the market today. A few of these are, Aspercreme, Bengay, Flexal, Mobisyl, and Sportscream.

Salicylates and counterirritants are for temporary relief only. These medications are also known as NSAIDs (non-steroidal anti-inflammatory drugs.) They are very useful and readily available for the reduction of arthritis pain at the source. The downside to these topical creams is that their effectiveness lessens over time. This occurs with over use. The body is adaptive by nature, so applying the creams and salves for a prolonged period causes the body to adapt to the burning or cooling sensation, so the medication becomes of little use. It is advised to seek the advice of your medical professional in the case of long-term care for arthritis.

3. COMMON TYPES OF ARTHRITIS AND TREATMENT OPTIONS

In addition to topical creams, there is a wide variety of other treatment options. Most of these treatment options are specific to the type of arthritis being treated. There are over 100 types of arthritis. Physicians determine treatment options based on type of arthritis being treated, the person's age, allergies the person may have, and any other medications being taken as to not counter-react or cause more complications. Here are some of the most common types of arthritis and treatment options.

- **Osteoarthritis**is also called "wear and tear arthritis." It is most common in older patients, usually over the age of 65. Over time, cartilage between joints breaks down, so instead of having that cushion between the joints bone meets bone and causes pain. Other causes of osteoarthritis are bone breakage, obesity, diabetes, inflammatory joint disease, and abnormalities in limb length, such as one leg being longer than the other. Genetics also plays a part in the development of osteoarthritis.

There are many medications for osteoarthritis. The most common are over the counter anti-inflammatory drugs, such as Advil, Alieve, Motrin, and Tylenol. These can be taken for pain relief relatively easily and pain relief lasts for hours. Sometimes these medications can even work up to twenty-four hours. Prolonged use of these medications need only be done under advisement (by) a physician. Your doctor may recommend a daily prescription treatment option. These treatments may offer better relief because they are of prescription strength and instead of taking multiple pills per day; you only need to remember to take one. Celebrex and Cymbalta are examples of these medications.

Usually, the last resort option for osteoarthritis sufferers is the most invasive. If cartilage has been broken down too much and the pain becomes too severe, surgery may be the only option for relief. This usually involves replacement of the entire joint. Most of these surgeries are done on the back, knee, or hip because most stress is placed on these joints. In addition to these surgeries follow up examinations must be performed, usually once or twice a year, to inspect the replaced joint. Recalls on metals used in joint replacement have recently made the monitoring of metal levels in the blood stream a necessity to maintain health after replacement surgery has occurred. A simple blood test is usually all that is needed to insure that these metal levels stay low. Any increase in metal levels can result in reoccurring pain. If pain does return and metal levels are elevated another surgery may have to be performed. If left unchecked, metal levels can rise to toxic levels and can result in toxic metal poisoning and death.

- **Rheumatoid Arthritis** unlike osteoarthritis is an autoimmune disease in which the body attacks its own tissues. This attack can lead to painful swelling and deforming of the hands or feet due to bone erosion. Whereas osteoarthritis is mainly seen in older patients, rheumatoid arthritis can attack anyone at any age. Most cases are seen in people above the age of 40, but this is not due to the wear and tear of joints. Women are at a higher risk of developing rheumatoid arthritis than men and genetics play a part in the development of the disease. Rheumatoid arthritis attacks the lining of the joint and it is said that 6% of the population of the United States suffers from rheumatoid arthritis.

Symptoms of rheumatoid arthritis include tender, warm, and swollen joints. Nodules may appear underneath the skin. A person may experience morning stiffness that can last for hours. Fatigue, fever, and weightless are also symptoms of rheumatoid arthritis. The disease will affect smaller joints, such as hands, first. If left unchecked larger joints and even organs can be attacked.

Treatment options vary depending on the severity of the rheumatoid arthritis. As with any arthritis the first option is anti-inflammatory creams and gels. Over-the-counter pain relievers such as Advil, Alieve, and Motrin are also recommended.

Steroids can be used to reduce inflammation and discomfort. Prednisone is one of the steroids that are commonly used. Steroids are not to be used for long periods and are to be gradually reduced in order to release the patient from the medication. Side effects from steroids can include severe lung infections, bone marrow suppression, and liver damage.

Disease-modifying antirheumatic drugs also known as DMARDs are another treatment option. These drugs are said to lower the progression of joint damage due to rheumatoid arthritis. These drugs include Trexall, Arava, Plaquenil, and Asulfidine. The side effects of these drugs can include severe lung infections, bone marrow suppression, and liver damage.

Immunosuppressants are said to bring the immune system back under control. Imvran, Asrasan, Neoral, Sandimmun and Gengraf are a few of these medications. The main side effect to these medications is an increased susceptibility to infection. Consultation with your doctor and consideration for this side effect is advised before starting on any of these medications.

TNF-alpha inhibitors help with the release of a natural substance in the body called tumor necrosis factor- alpha. This substance is an anti-inflammatory that can reduce swelling and inflammation in joints. TNF- alpha inhibitors are Enbrel, Remicade, Humira, Simponi, and Cimzia. These medications also can have severe side effects. These side effects may include, but are not limited to, an increased risk of infection, hair loss, nausea, and diarrhea.

The most practical form of relief from rheumatoid arthritis is therapy. A nurse can show you simple movements, stretches, and exercises that may reduce the swelling, inflammation, and pain associated with rheumatoid arthritis. A nurse can also give you tips on different ways of doing things in which you will not have to use painful joints. There are also many new inventions that can make it easier to use everyday items with less strain on sore joints.

As with osteoarthritis, surgery is the last option. There are a few types of surgeries associated with rheumatoid arthritis. The joint may have to be completely removed in order for full relief to occur. There is also an option to just have the tendon repaired if it has ruptured due to inflammation. Joint fusion may also be recommended if the other options are unavailable or impossible to do.

• **Gouty Arthritis** occurs when there are crystal deposits of uric acid in the joints. This is the most painful of all the types of arthritis. Gouty arthritis accounts for about 5% of all arthritis cases. Although, it is painful it is one of the most treatable. Gout is most common in men and very rare in children. Gout most commonly shows up in the big toe first, but can also affect the ankles, feet, fingers, elbows, and wrists.

There are four stages of gouty arthritis.

1. **Asymptomatic Hyeruricemia**- This stage requires no treatment. It is when uric acid levels are elevated in the bloodstream.

2. **Acute Gouty Arthritis**- At this stage crystal deposits of uric acid have been detected and can lead to attacks.

3. **Intercritical**- In this stage there are no symptoms between gout attacks.

4. **Chronic Tophaceous Gout**- If this stage is reached; permanent damage has already been done. With proper care from a physician, a slow but rewarding recovery can be achieved.

Gouty arthritis can cause the affected joints to become inflamed. Anti-inflammatory, such as Advil can help to manage the pain. It is advised that a person suffering from a gout attack not take aspirin as aspirin can cause a rise in uric acid levels. For chronic gout treatment, your doctor may recommend a prescription medication. Some of these medications are Colchicine-probenecid, Kystexxa intravenous, and pegloticase intravenous.

- **Pseudogout** is also known as false gout. Pseudogout occurs when calcium pyrophosphate crystals form in the cartilage of the joint. Sudden pain will occur when these crystals are released into the joint fluid. The cause for these calcium crystals is unknown and attacks only last between 5 and 12 days even when no treatment is being applied. This form of arthritis attacks men and women equally and is more common in people over the age of 60.

Symptoms of pseudogout include swollen joints that are warm to the touch, intense joint pain that comes on without warning, severe tenderness around joints, and the skin around joints may appear red or even purple.

There are many medications to treat pseudogout. These medications require a prescription so a consultation with your physician is required. A few of these medications are Medrol, Dex Pac, Pediapred, Flopred, and Prednisone Intersol.

• **Lupus Arthritis** is different from traditional arthritis, but has some of the same symptoms and is treated in the same way. Unlike typical arthritis, lupus arthritis does not affect the spine or the neck. Flair ups can be very painful and symptoms include swollen and painful joints, excessive fatigue, and a rash in the shape of a butterfly on the cheek and nose. Other symptoms include hair loss, sensitivity to light, pain in the chest, mouth or nose sores, and pale or purple fingers and toes.

The cause of lupus arthritis is unknown, but there are many treatment options.

1. **Steroids**- In the forms of creams or pills, steroids are used in low doses to treat low to moderate lupus arthritis.

2. **Plaqueril**- This drug is also for low to moderate lupus arthritis and is a daily medicine that helps prevent lupus arthritis flare-ups.

3. **Cytoxan**- Mostly used in chemotherapy this drug is used for lupus arthritis when the disease becomes severe enough that it is affecting the kidneys and brain.

4. **Imuran**- This drug is usually used in organ transplant patients to ensure that the organ is accepted by the body. Imuran is only used in serious cases of lupus arthritis.

5. **Rheumatrex**- Another chemotherapy drug, rheumatrex reduces the number of abnormal B cells that are common in lupus arthritis patients.

6. **Cellcept**- This is another drug used in organ transplants that has shown improvements in lupus arthritis sufferers.

7. **Rituxan**- For serious cases of lupus arthritis. This biologic agent is only used as a last resort when all else fails.

Lupus arthritis most often affects women. Women are 10 times more likely to suffer from lupus arthritis than men are. Studies have also shown that lupus effects people of African, Asian, and Native American decent. This very treatable form of arthritis offers its victims a fighting chance. If doctor's orders are followed and the disease is kept in check, a person diagnosed with lupus arthritis can expect full life expectancy with little aggravation.

- **Psoriatic Arthritis** is only in patients that have a previous history of psoriasis. About 80% of patients will have psoriasis for decades before psoriatic arthritis occurs. The disease comes on in the same ways as other forms of arthritis. Painful swelling of the joints is the first sign. Many times, it attacks the fingers first. One finger will become inflamed and very painful. The infected finger will often double in size and resemble a sausage. Unlike other forms of arthritis, psoriatic arthritis is rare and can affect the eyes, kidneys, lung lining, and in rare cases, the aorta. Inflammation in cartilage and tendons can also occur.

Psoriatic arthritis comes in five forms:

1. **Symmetric-** This form occurs when the same joint or joints is affected on either side of the body. If untreated, this form of psoriatic arthritis can cause deformities. The good news is that this form is also the most mild if treated properly.

2. **Asymmetric-** Unlike symmetric, which affects both sides of the body, asymmetric can affect any joint at any

time. It can lead to deformities', but this is unlikely if the disease is treated in the proper manner.

3. Distal Interphalangeal Predominant (DIP) - In this form of arthritis, the joint closest to fingernail and toenails is affected. With this form of the disease the joints become inflamed and changes in the nail can occur. DIP accounts for only 5% of all cases of psoriatic arthritis.

4. Spondylitis- Affecting only about 5% of all psoriatic arthritis sufferers, this form attacks the spinal cord. Stiffness in the neck, shoulders, and back is common. Movement can become difficult, but like with most other forms of arthritis, with proper treatment, symptoms can be reduced.

5. Mutilans- This form of psoriatic arthritis is the rarest and worst form. It accounts for less than 5% of all psoriatic arthritis cases. Attacks come on quickly, with rapid deterioration of the joints, resulting in deformities'. Mutilans usually affects small joints but has been known to cause back and neck pain.

With only about 2% of the entire Caucasian population suffering from psoriasis, this form of arthritis is very rare and usually easily treated. As with most forms of arthritis, psoriatic arthritis is treated with anti-inflammatory drugs. These drugs come in the form of creams and gels for the first stages and pills, such as Reumatrex and Trexall, for the more advanced cases.

- **Enteropathic Arthritis** is a form of arthritis that occurs in people with inflammatory bowel disease, Crohns's disease, and ulcerative colitis. Most cases affect those with inflammatory bowel disease. About 20% of patients with inflammatory bowel disease will develop enteropathic arthritis. Your doctor will run tests to determine the presents of the arthritis. They typically test for anemia and elevated levels of inflammation.

Treatment of enteropathic arthritis is different from that of other arthritis treatments. The other diseases that are associated with enteropathic arthritis must be considered so the use of NSAIDs that can typically ease the pain of arthritis are not recommended because they can cause aggravation of inflammatory bowel disease. Treatment for this form of arthritis is typically done with the use of anit-TNF drugs. These drugs effectively treat the arthritis without aggravating the other disease. Anti-TNF drugs include Humiria, Cimzia and Remicade.

• **Infectious Arthritis** can affect anyone at any age. Infectious arthritis occurs when a joint becomes infected. The infections can enter the body in the form of a germ. These germs can come in the form of bacteria, fungus, or a virus.

Bacteria are the most likely cause of infectious arthritis. It can come from bacterial infections such as gonorrhea, strep throat, pneumonia, tuberculosis, spirochetes, and homophilus.

Viruses that can bring cases of infectious arthritis are mumps, mono, and infectious forms of hepatitis.

Fungi associated with infectious arthritis can come from the soil, bird droppings, and even roses.

Diagnosis is made by taking a fluid sample from the joint that is infected. Doctors prefer to hold off on antibiotics unless the patient is at a critical level. This is because the cause of the infectious arthritis is impossible to determine once antibiotics are in the system. Patients are often put into the hospital in order for fluid to be drained from the infected joint. Blood tests are also usually done to determine the source of the infection.

Infectious arthritis is usually not a lifetime disease if treated quickly. Within 24 hours of the infection beginning permanent damage can occur, so medical attention needs to be sought immediately if abnormal swelling occurs after an operation

- **Hemorrhagic Arthritis** is when blood is in the joint. Risk factors associated with hemorrhagic arthritis are conditions that cause trauma to the body, especially trauma associated with excessive bleeding. Sickle cell anemia and hemophilia are also risk factors.

This type of arthritis is treated in much the same way as other forms of the disease. NSAIDs may be recommended to relieve pain. Hemorrhagic arthritis is a form of arthritis that is not serious and is treated relatively easily.

In every type of arthritis, there is one common denominator, age. Every one of us is going to get older and we must take care of our bodies so they can last as long as possible. You may not believe that there is anything that can be done about the effects of getting older, but there are. We can spend our early years eating what we want without the risk of much of anything because when your body is young, it is able to fight off infection with no problem. As we get older if not properly cared for, our bodies tend to begin to break down. Joints need lubrication to function properly. Most people, when they think of hydration, will grab whatever sugary drink happens to be in arms reach. This practice will put you at higher risk for developing arthritis. Proper lubrication of the joints begins with water. Water is one of the basic needs of human existence. Lack of water affects every organ, muscle, and bone in the body. With our bodies being primarily made up of water we need more than we get. Along with getting enough water there are other foods which can significantly reduce the risk of arthritis and help with the pain of arthritis in someone who has already been diagnosed with the condition.

4. FOODS THAT CAN HELP ARTHRITIS SUFFERERS

The advancements in pharmaceutical medication in recent years have been mind-blowing. Advances in medicine have produced cures and remedies for diseases that have plagued human kind for decades. These advancements in modern medicine are wonderful, no doubt, but what did people do before all the chemically made drugs were available to the masses? For one, people were much more active in the past than they are now. Our ancestor's days were not filled with hours spent in front of a television or checking mindlessly their mobile devices sucking up useless information on which celebrity is doing outrageous things in Hollywood. People had to survive. There was no going to a fast food chain and picking up something high in fat and calories to eat just because you did not feel like cooking. There was a garden on every piece of land occupied by a family. Jobs were primarily farming and the farming was done without the use of harmful chemicals. People ate better back then. They ate cleaner. Unless the family had an animal that could be killed, meat was a luxury. Most of the meat that was eaten was chicken or fish because chickens were readily available and cheap and most pieces of property contained a water source that provided great fishing. Back then, people only took from the land what would be used. They did not rob the earth of everything it had to give in order for the family to have abundance. People treated the land with respect because it was their life source.

The bottom line is that food is and always will be the best source of medication. Natural foods are filled with all the nutrients necessary to control the symptoms of many diseases including arthritis. Here is a list of foods that can help with the pain associated with arthritis. It is not advised to stop using medications prescribed by your doctor, but these foods are a tool that can be used to aid in the prevention of arthritis symptoms.

Salmon has a variety of uses in many different illnesses. For arthritis sufferers the Omega 3 fatty acids that aid in the prevention of inflammation spreading chemicals. It is suggested that arthritis sufferers eat at least 1 gram of Omega 3 fatty acids per day. Salmon contains 1.5 grams for every 4oz. serving. Salmon also contains vitamin D that aids in the relief of soreness and swelling.

Extra Virgin Olive Oil contains olecanthal. Olecanthal is a substance that helps to block the enzymes that are involved in the inflammation that is the main cause of arthritis pain. Ibuprofen is used by most arthritis sufferers to lessen inflammation and pain. Extra virgin olive oil contains 1/10 of a dose of ibuprofen for every 3 tablespoons used. This is not to say that extra virgin olive oil should be used to replace ibuprofen because extra virgin olive oil does have a high calorie content, but adding a little into your diet every day as a preventative will reduce the reliance on anti-inflammatory drugs.

Brazil Nuts are tasty as well as helpful. They contain selenium that is a mineral that aids in clearing out free radicals that are known to damage cells. It is suggested that an arthritis sufferer take 55 – 200 micrograms of selenium per day. Brazil nuts contain 272 micrograms in about every four nuts. Therefore, even if they are not your favorite food, it is not that hard to eat four nuts per day in order to maintain proper health.

Onions are both a flavor additive and readily available in many forms. Onions are easily added to almost any food and are available in an infinite number of varieties to satisfy any palette. Whether you like a strong onion flavor or prefer the more mild varieties there is an onion out there for everyone. All varieties are good for arthritis patients for the simple fact that onions contain Quercetin. Quercetin is an antioxidant that has been proven to inhibit anti-inflammatory chemicals in the body.

Cherries are often overlooked for their medicinal properties. I am not talking about the jar of maraschino cherries we buy to put on ice cream. I am referring to the fresh tart cherries that are available in the produce section of any grocery store. The pigment in cherries, which gives them that vibrant deep red color, contains authocyanins that help in the reduction of inflammation in the body. It is suggested that a person suffering with arthritis try to add ½ cup of tart cherries or an oz of cherry juice to their diet on a daily basis to help with inflammation.

Green Tea contains epigallocatechin- 3 – gallate (EGCG). This is an effective anti-inflammatory and it is suggested that arthritis patients strive to drink 3 to 4 cups of caffeinated green tea daily to aid in the prevention of inflammation. The caffeinated variety is suggested because it contains more helpful nutrients than decaffeinated tea.

Beans are a meat substitute as well as a natural muscle relaxer. Beans are available in a wide variety of shapes, colors, and textures. They are easy to add to mostly any dish and have the added benefit of being high in calcium that helps strengthen bones.

Flax seed in raw form must be ground in order for health benefits to be released. In arthritis patients, flaxseed has been proven to reduce inflammation and swelling, as well as, relieve stiffness and joint pain. As I stated before, joints need lubrication in order for them to move correctly. Flaxseed is full of oils that offer this lubrication. It is suggested that taking 3 grams of flaxseed in ground form or 1 to 3 tablespoons in the form of flaxseed oil will help relieve arthritis symptoms. Flaxseed is also a good source for Omega- 3 fatty acids for those who do not particularly enjoy fish.

Soya beans are available in a variety of products these days, but all soya bean products are not created equal. To enjoy the anti-inflammatory properties of soya beans they must be consumed in the least processed form as possible. Edamame, soya milk, and tofu are the forms of soya beans that will be most beneficial in the fight against arthritis.

Whole Grains have been everywhere in recent years. The processing of grains to make products such as flour, strip the grains of needed nutrients. Whole grains reduce C reactive protein levels that inhibit inflammation. Switching from single grain products to whole grain is a simple way to reduce sugar in your diet and help with arthritis symptoms.

Tomatoes are a very versatile ingredient. They can be added to almost any dish and offer a sweet taste without having to add any sugar. The vibrant red color makes an ordinary recipe come alive. Tomatoes offer high levels of lycopene which, you guessed it, lessens inflammation. As opposed to other vegetables and fruits, which are to be eaten raw in order to gain the most nutrients, tomatoes contain more lycopene when cooked.

Beets are an ingredient that children have been turning their noses up at for decades. They stain everything they touch and yes, they do have anti-inflammatory qualities. Beets are packed with antioxidants that aid in the reduction of inflammation.

Walnuts are another nut high in Omega- 3 fatty acids. Walnuts actually contain the highest number of Omega-3 fatty acids. In fact, only ¼ cup of walnuts will provide you with 94.6% of the daily-recommended value of these fatty acids. Therefore, those of you opposed to fish can still get the nutrients you need to treat the inflammation associated with arthritis.

Cashews are unlike the other nuts for use in arthritis care. These nuts are rich in copper and magnesium. Copper controls free radicals that can do major damage to the bodies' tissues. Cashews contain 40% of the recommended daily intake of copper. Magnesium is paramount in maintaining bone density. About 22% of the daily-recommended intake of magnesium can be found in cashews.

Ginger is a much-underused root. The medicinal properties of ginger are vast when it comes to the treatment of certain diseases. Specifically, for the treatment of arthritis ginger is a natural pain reliever and an anit-inflammatory. Ginger is offered in a variety of forms to fit the needs of any person. The raw form of ginger can be found in the produce section and is most effective in treating pain and inflammation caused by arthritis. The root can be sliced off and boiled to make a healthy tea. It can also be found in canned or dried form and can be added to most desserts.

Apples are a powerhouse of nutrients that treat a large range of ailments. For the treatment of arthritis, apples contain boron. Boron has been shown to be an effective pain reliever. Apple cider vinegar is of particular interest because of the shelf life and the ease of taking it. A reduction in pain will be noticed after a few months of mixing 2 tablespoons of apple cider vinegar with 8 oz. of water and drinking the mixture 2 or 3 times per day. In addition, a bath in apple cider vinegar mixed with water helps relieve soreness.

Broccoli has been shown to be an extremely effective food in both the prevention and treatment of arthritis. Broccoli contains sulforaphane that offers strong antioxidant properties. Antioxidants kill harmful free radical preventing them from killing healthy cells. It is the harmful effects of free radicals that are believed to be a major cause of arthritis.

Pumpkin Seeds are not just the discarded waste from carving pumpkins, but also a very effective muscle and nerve relaxer. Pumpkin seeds are high in magnesium that also strengthens bones for better circulation. Just ½ cup of pumpkin seeds provides 46.1% of daily-recommended magnesium, 28.7% that of iron, 52% of manganese, 24% of copper, 16.9% of protein, and 17.1% of zinc.

These are just a small number of the foods that may help the reduction of symptoms associated with arthritis. On the contrary, there are also foods that need to be avoided when arthritis is a factor. Fried foods can increase symptoms of arthritis by aiding in the inflammation of joints. Sugary snacks are also contributors to the flare up of arthritis symptoms. More of these foods include those high in salt, dairy products, alcoholic beverages, foods high in carbohydrates and red meat. Frozen and processed foods should also be avoided. Even though a particular frozen food says that it is healthier for you does not mean it is a good idea to eat it. Some frozen dinners claim that they are low in calories, but if you actually look at the ingredients, these foods contain a much higher level of sodium. They may be lower in fat but not healthier.

In the search for a healthier lifestyle with less arthritis pain, fresh is always the best option. Canned goods have been pasteurized to increase shelf life, but in the pasteurization process much of the nutrients are lost. When heat is applied to most foods many of the nutrients escapes with the steam. It is best to cook vegetables and fruits for the shortest time possible in order to maintain the nutrients at their highest peak.

Although there is no cure for arthritis, it is possible to eat your way to a reduction in arthritis symptoms. Eating healthy takes dedication and a positive outlook. Look for recipes that use a variety of good foods along with a variety of color. People eat with their eyes first so preparing beautiful dishes with varieties of colors offer a feast for the eyes. Get the entire family involved. It is important to have support when making a lifestyle change to eat better. With a supportive family, it is easier to stay on track and it is also important to have accountability.

Children especially, do a very good job of holding their parents accountable for things they say. Tell them the dangers of unhealthy eating and explain why some foods are good and some foods are bad. We all want our children to grow up and be better than what we, ourselves, have been. A child that is well trained on the subject of healthy eating may stray from teachings as they grow, but will always have that base to come back to. There are also many cases where children who grow up in a home with high standards of healthy eating and continue that lifestyle without straying. They have adapted their tastes to certain foods and never developed a taste for fast food or processed foods. There is a trend lately of entire families giving up sugar of any kind. In one particular case, the whole family vowed to give up sugar for one entire year. They allowed themselves only one sugary treat each month. After two months of sugar deprivation, the family began to not enjoy the sweet monthly treat at all. After 6 months, the sweet treat began to cause headaches in the family, so they eventually just stopped eating it altogether. The family felt better and even looked better. Everyone was more active and enjoyed a better quality of family time.

Sugar acts in many ways like a drug. In modern society, sugar is everywhere and therefore people have become accustomed to eating much more than they should. In cases, like above, where people purposely deprive their bodies of sugar the body will go through a series of withdrawals. These withdrawals mimic the same symptoms that a drug addict exhibits when in rehab. Mood swings can occur for a while when people resist sugar. Some people will even develop "the shakes". Sugar is an addictive substance. It releases dopamine in our bodies causing us to feel good. Sugar is not the only problem when it comes to arthritis, but controlling one aspect at a time will allow an arthritis sufferer to become aware of things that can trigger an arthritis attack. Being aware of these triggers is the first step in controlling arthritis symptoms and getting a grip on the disease.

In addition to children and family living in the home, let your co-workers and extended family support you. It is important to surround yourself with as many positive influences as possible. It is very easy to fall into old habits of eating greasy sugary foods because they are readily available. Do not get upset if someone makes a mention that, a particular food you are eating is not good for you. Be happy and encouraged that so many people care for you and want you to be around for a long time. Bad habits do not go away overnight; they must be acknowledged and cultivated into good habits.

5.   FREE WAYS TO SEEK ARTHRITIS RELIEF

Pharmaceuticals are always available for arthritis relief. Doctors are quick to write prescriptions for whatever symptom is bothering the patient. The problem is that doctors are expensive and the prescriptions that are prescribed are sometimes as much as a house payment every month. Without insurance, arthritis prescriptions can be impossible to obtain. There are free ways to gain arthritis relief. The main one is exercise. Movement can be difficult when arthritis symptoms flare, but it is essential in relieving the pain. There are certain exercises that can reduce pain and discomfort.

Morning Stretches- After great night sleep, it is tempting to jump up quickly and get the day going. If you are like most people it is even more tempting to just stay in bed and hit the snooze button. Neither of these are a good idea when arthritis relief is the main goal. To start the day off right, sit up slowly and place your feet on the floor. Take 10 deep breaths. The deep breaths will stretch your lungs and make breathing easier. Deep breathing is also good for asthma sufferers and it is a good idea to do this exercise a few times a day. Next, place your hands on your knees and slowly rise off the bed to a standing position. Slowly bring your arms above your head and stretch. Hold this for a few seconds and then bring your arms back to your sides. Relax your body and slowly roll your head from one side to the other. Stretch your neck muscles as much as you feel comfortable. Next, place your hands on your hips and stretch your upper body from side to side. Do this a few times and then bend over to stretch and try to touch your toes. These stretches will help with flexibility and movement throughout the day. They will also help your mind wake up and be ready for the day.

Finger Stretches- Arthritis attacks smaller joints first. Because these joints are so small, they can deteriorate faster than larger joints in the body. Finger stretches are a great and easy way to maintain movements in finger joints. Extend your arm out from your body in front of you with your palm facing up. Starting with the thumb, touch your palm 10 times. Do this with all other fingers one at a time and with the other hand. After all fingers have been stretched, extend one arm in front of you again and use the other hand to pull your fingers back stretching the wrist. Repeat this with the other hand.

Walking- It may be difficult starting out, but walking every day will ensure joints get the exercise they need in order to stay healthy. Start slow, walk down the drive way and back a few times. As days go by you can increase the distance and pace of your walk. Walking the same place every day may become stale and boring so change it up every so often. Walk at the park or if weather becomes a problem find an indoor place to walk. If you live close to town, walk to town instead of driving for simple errands. When walking, incorporate your arms so that all muscles get a workout. Get people involved with your walking routine. Invite people to walk with you. Many people find that they walk for longer if there is someone there to talk with.

Lifting Weights - This is not to suggest that a massive body building endeavor is in order. Lifting small weights and offering a little resistance can help with joint health. Again, start slow when beginning weight lifting exercises. The goal is joint health not to push your body to the point of injury. A two-pound weight is a good starting point. Do reps of 10 at a time. Start with your arms lifting the weight out to the side, above your head, and behind your neck. Start with one arm and then go to the other to give each arm rest between reps. Weight can also be added to legs. Add a five-pound weight to each leg and do simple leg lifts. Weight training can be done every day. It is important to listen to your body and not push yourself too hard. If pain gets too bad, take a day off. It will take time for your body to adjust to weight training.

Tai Chi - This exercise is practiced in many Asian countries and has also, in recent years, become popular around the world. Tai Chi involves a series of slow, precise movements. These slow movements make it easy for arthritis sufferers to do these exercises. There is no need to go to a class to learn the art of Tai Chi. There are many websites and books that can be used for instruction.

Yoga - This form of exercise is excellent for people suffering from arthritis pain. Yoga is a series of poses that allow you to stretch various parts of the body. These poses are very easy to do and offer a low impact workout with a relaxing effect on the body. Yoga encourages deep breathing during the exercises that helps to calm and increase blood flow to the brain. In this process, your own body is used for resistance so there is no special equipment to buy. Yoga poses are easily found on the internet or in books from a library.

Off the Wall Pushups - These are very effective for people who are having arthritis issues in their hands and wrists. It offers enough resistance to exercise wrist muscles without having all of your body weight on your wrists like with traditional pushups. Place your hands on the wall and step back as far as you feel comfortable. The farther you stand back, the more resistance will be in the exercise. Push against the wall and do as many pushups as you feel comfortable with.

Swimming - You do not need a membership to a fitness club with a fancy pool to enjoy a good swim. Find a friend with a pool that you can swim laps in. Swimming offers a great workout with very little pressure on the joints. Swimming laps in a pool will use all the muscles in your body. After swimming your laps, move to the deep end and tread water for as long as you can hold out. Treading water works your lower body muscles without putting pressure on the joints like running and walking will.

Doing any exercise will improve the overall health of your joints and your body. It is important to find a reason to stand up and walk around at least once every hour. Sitting still will make your joints more stiff and prone to arthritis flare-ups.

In addition to exercise, there are many other ways to seek arthritis relief without paying a dime. One of the most effective ways is to simply drink water. Water is an essential part of life. Without water, life is impossible. Water makes up most of our bodies. Lubrication of joints is essential for arthritis relief. Drinking the proper amount of water will allow your joints to get the lubrication they require to make movement easier. Water can also be used in ways, apart from drinking it, to help alleviate arthritis pain. A warm bath is often the best remedy to relax sore muscles. Soaking in a bath for 20 or 30 minutes is the perfect way to end a hard day. Warm water will surround the body; will melt stress and strain away.

Massage is also a way to alleviate arthritis pressure. I am not talking about spending enormous amounts of money on a professional massage. I am simply saying that rubbing your hands with baby oil and massaging joints can alleviate pain caused by an arthritis flare up. Massage joints with just a small amount of pressure and use a circular pattern. This circular motion causes the joint or muscle to relax and the pain will, most often, go away.

There are many ways to find arthritis relief

without breaking the bank. Whichever option you decide to use, be sure you are comfortable with it. Do not do any exercise or home remedy that you do not understand or that makes you nervous. You know your body better than any other person does and you know your limits. It is advised that you consult your doctor. If by some chance, you cannot make it to the doctor or you do not have a regular physician, talk to a local pharmacist. They are a great source for information regarding remedies and over the counter medications. Pharmacists are usually only used to fill prescriptions, but in fact a pharmacist is sometimes the best free source for medical advice.

ARTHRITIS

6. DAILY TIPS TO GAIN CONTROL OF ARTHRITIS PAIN

There are many tricks and tips to controlling arthritis pain. One of the most prevalent is to not overstrain muscles and joints. Anything that can be done to reduce strain on joints and muscles will make an impact of arthritis relief. Gaining control of arthritis pain means taking charge to prevent arthritis symptoms so a flare up does not occur.

Making meals can put stress and strain on anyone. Making meals when your joints are inflamed makes the task almost impossible. Invest in devices that make life easier. There are many products that make doing things around the house simple for arthritis sufferers. The use of a jar or bottle opener offers a simple solution to reduce strain on joints. The use of a chopper instead of a knife to cut vegetables can make preparing dinner a little easier. Using an electric mixer to blend ingredients instead of a whisk can put less strain on joints. Re organizes your kitchen to make things that are used most often easier to reach. An organized kitchen produces fewer accidents. Place heavier objects on lower shelves to keep from having to reach up and bring down those heavy objects. Picking an object up to place it on the counter is usually less strain on the joints.

Reorganize your clothes as well. This may seem a little strange, but if you have trouble opening the drawers of a dresser, you may want to hang clothes in the closet. Instead of having to open the dresser drawers to take out clothes, you can simply pull on the clothes and they often fall right off the hanger. Also, avoid using button up shirts. Trying to button up a shirt during an arthritis flare up can be frustrating and painful.

Ask for help when needed. Generally, people have an, "I can do it myself," attitude when they need help. There is no shame in asking someone for help. It is much better to ask someone for help in doing a seemingly small task than asking someone to help you get to the hospital because you were stubborn and hurt yourself. Family and friends will be happy to help with anything you need. If mowing the lawn becomes too much, let one of the younger people in the family take the task over. If certain cleaning tasks become a problem around the house, call someone over to assist. There is no need to hurt yourself or overstrain your muscles to impress others with an immaculate house. No one is superman. We all need help from time to time.

The use of essential oils is also a way to take charge in the fight against arthritis pain. These oils have been used for centuries to aid in the treatments of many ailments. They can be a little expensive, but very little oil goes a long way. Here are five essential oils that can be used to treat arthritis pain.

Lavender Oil - This oil is a major player if you are seeking forms of natural healing. The uses for lavender oil are endless. If only one oil is to be gotten, this is it. Specifically in the treatment of arthritis, lavender oil offers anti-inflammatory properties and can be applied to any affected area. Lavender oil has also been known to be a great sleep aid. Rest is essential in the treatment of arthritis. Relaxed muscles are happy muscles.

Marjoram Oil - This oil can be applied directly to ailing muscles and can also be used on pressure point in the feet that have been historically used to relieve all sorts of disorders. Marjoram oil helps reduce muscle spasms and relieve stiff joints.

Eucalyptus Oil - This oil is already in many over the counter arthritis remedies, but in its raw form is a very effective anti-inflammatory. It can also be applied to the affected area or applied to pressure points.

Rosemary Oil - The herb form is used most often in dishes to offer a sweet aroma to different types of meat. In pure oil form, this herb is used for natural pain relief and as an anti-inflammatory.

Peppermint Oil - Historically used for many ailments from foot odor to dandruff, peppermint oil offers arthritis sufferers another natural anti-inflammatory.

These five oils can be used by themselves or as a group to relieve the aches and pains associated with arthritis. The only drawback to using essential oils is the time it takes to adjust your body to them. With modern medicine, relief can come within fifteen minutes of applying or taking the medicine. Essential oils take time to fully absorb into your body to become effective. It can take several weeks for you to feel the effects of these essential oils. The major plus to these oils is the lack of side effects. Over the counter creams, pills, or other arthritis remedies can have a number of side effects and are loaded with chemicals. As these over the counter remedies are highly effective in treating arthritis you do not always know what exactly is going into your body. Essential oils are strait forward natural ingredients.

What you need to know about arthritis and supplements

Supplements aid in providing the body with the essential nutrients it needs to function correctly. If you have ever stood in the supplement isle at any store, you realize that there are many. Confusion can set in quickly when deciding on what supplement is right for you. One may offer relief in one area of importance, but be a bad idea for another ailment you may be suffering with. Some of these supplements cannot be found in any foods and can only be found in supplement form. Supplements are not controlled by the food and drug administration so their use is strictly at the discretion of the consumer. Here is a list of arthritis supplements that will help in your quest for arthritis relief.

Glucosamine aids in preventing the worsening of cartilage. With healthy cartilage, joints move more freely. Studies have also shown that glucosamine aids in the building of cartilage. There are some side effects associated with glucosamine. This supplement is derived from shellfish and any person with a shellfish allergy should consult their doctor before beginning the use of glucosamine. It is also advised that any woman who is pregnant or breastfeeding consult their doctor before taking this supplement. Glucosamine can affect the absorption of insulin into the body so anyone using insulin should use caution. This supplement can also cause diarrhea, nausea, indigestion, and heartburn.

Chondroitin helps to keep cartilage healthy. It can also help with joint pain and can reduce inflammation. Side effects include mild stomach pain and nausea. Pregnant or breastfeeding women are urged to consult their physician before taking chondroitin. It has also been shown to cause an increase in asthma symptoms and been linked to causing prostate cancer.

SAMe or S- adenosyl-Lmethionineis a substance made naturally in the body. In a supplement form SAMs acts like NSAIDs. It was found by mistake when physicians used it to treat depression, the patients bragged at how much better their joints symptoms were feeling. So quite by accident, a new arthritis remedy was discovered. There are many side effects with the supplement form of SAMe. These include insomnia, dry mouth, sweating, vomiting, gas, and dizziness. SAMe has also been known to make bipolar disorder and Parkinson's worse. It is also recommended that a patient should stop taking SAMe 2 weeks before any surgery as the supplement can cause complications.

MSM or Methylsulfonylmethane is a chemical found in animals, plants, and humans. It has been proven to help form connective tissue. The side effects of MSM include headache, bloating, diarrhea, itching, and can worsen symptoms in allergy sufferers.

Omega 3 Fatty acids have already been discussed previously for their anti-inflammatory properties. This substance that is naturally found in fish is also available as a supplement for those who do not like the flavor of fish. Omega 3 fatty acid supplements should not be taken if you are on blood thinners or already taking anti-inflammatory drugs. The only real side effects associated with Omega 3 fatty acids are upset stomach and diarrhea.

Vitamin C, which is found in many natural

substances, is also available in a supplement. The supplement form of vitamin C aids in the building of connective tissue in the body. The side effects of this supplement are quite few. Taking too much vitamin C while pregnant can cause problems with your newborn. Anyone who is to undergo angioplasty is advised against taking vitamin C as it can cause complications in the procedure. In diabetes patients, taking too much vitamin C can raise blood sugar levels. It can also increase kidney stones in people who are already at high risk for getting kidney stones. Too much vitamin C can also cause complications in people with sickle cell disease.

Ginger as was discussed earlier is an effective pain reliever in its natural form. The same is said about the supplement form of ginger. There are side effects of ginger in the supplement form. These are heartburn, stomachache, and diarrhea. Other risks include an increased risk for miscarriage and an increased risk for bleeding during surgery. Studies have also shown that the supplement form of ginger can lower blood sugar to dangerous levels in diabetes patients and can worsen many heart conditions.

Turmeric is another natural substance that science has turned into a supplement. The supplement of turmeric has proven to be a very effective pain reliever. The risks of turmeric in supplement form include upset stomach, nausea, diarrhea, and dizziness. There is also a risk to pregnant women and those with gallbladder issues. It is also recommended that patients who are undergoing any type of surgery should not take turmeric as it can cause severe bleeding.

Bromelain is a supplement that is used to alleviate soreness. It is also very effective at reducing inflammation. With a risk of bleeding, it is recommended that anyone undergoing surgery should discontinue use of bromelain for two weeks before surgery. People with certain allergies should avoid taking bromelain. These allergies include papain, celery, grass, cypress, pineapple, wheat, fennel, and carrot.

Devil's Claw is a supplement that reduces inflammation and pain in arthritis patients. This is available in a natural form, but in supplement form, there are side effects. An increase of gallstones may occur. Those with stomach ulcers are advised not to take devil's claw as it can increase stomach problems. It can increase heat rate so those with heart problems are strongly cautioned. Devil's claw has also been known to lower blood sugar levels so those with diabetes should take that into consideration.

As you can see, supplements can be complicated and each one has its own set of risks. As with any medical endeavor, it is strongly advised to seek answers from a medical professional. These and other supplements can help as well as harm so it is important for you and your doctor to discuss risk factors before supplements are taken. With the right advice from the right medical professional supplements can be a very effective tool in the prevention of arthritis symptoms.

7. CAYENNE PEPPER AND ARTHRITIS RELIEF

When it comes to arthritis, health doctors believe they have a handle on how to treat symptoms. As there have been many advancements in the treatment of arthritis by modern medicines the fact is that treatment for the disorder has been around for centuries. Nature is full of substances with healing properties. The cayenne pepper is one of these natural healers.

When settlers arrived in America, they were out of their element, in a sense, and had to rely on the Native Americans to show them how to live in this new land. The Native Americans taught the settlers how to cultivate the land and grow the necessary food in order to survive in this very strange environment. As the settlers and the Native Americans began to work together, the settlers noticed the Native Americans consuming these fiery hot chilies known today as cayenne pepper. The settlers were astonished that the Native Americans were not crying out in pain from these tiny infernos. The Native Americans were eating these peppers much like we today would eat an apple or an orange. It was just every day fare to them. They knew something way back then that modern medicine is only during this century began to discover. Cayenne pepper is a medicinal substance that can treat a plethora of illnesses. The Native Americans realized that consuming this pepper every day acted as a preventative for many aches and pains. We think we have it all figured out, but our ancestors deserve more credit than we have given them.

After being schooled by the Native Americans, the pepper was brought back to the West Indies and later found its way into many other countries. Europe began using cayenne in the treatment of muscle spasms. Chinese herbalists use cayenne as an effective treatment for frostbite. The Japanese employ cayenne pepper as an appetite suppressant. In the 1800s, American herbalist and Godfather of modern herbal use in America, Samuel Thomson, used cayenne in the treatment of many cardiovascular disorders. He also used the pepper to treat other disorders from asthma to ulcers. This form of herbal medicine has been used around the world for centuries and modern medicine has finally taken notice. Many medicines today contain cayenne pepper in some form or another.

In raw form, the cayenne pepper looks very small and insignificant. The spicy pepper has been used as a flavor additive to add punch to many regional cuisines. It is traditionally used in western style dishes to give them their signature spice. This hollow fruit is grown in tropical and subtropical climates. When cayenne peppers are ripe, they are red, yellow, or orange in color. They can be used in recipes from raw form, but most forms of cayenne come in the form of cayenne pepper. It is easily added to a variety of recipes. Traditionally cayenne has been used in main course cooking, but in recent years, a surge of desserts have begun using the pepper. It started as a trend, but has since grown into a way to add cayenne in to all aspects of diet. Chocolate is of particular interest when it comes to adding cayenne to desserts. The heat is, at first, masked by the sweet taste of the chocolate, but as the chocolate melts on the tongue, the release of spicy cayenne wakes up the taste buds causing the consumer to enjoy many more flavors the chocolate has to offer. These new flavors are often dulled by simply the sweet flavor. Cayenne brings out the complexity of the ingredient.

The active ingredient in cayenne pepper is capsaicin. This is the substance that gives cayenne pepper its spice. The effects of capsaicin have probably already been felt by you without your even knowing it. Capsaicin is found in any spicy peppers. If you have ever cut hot peppers, forgot to wash your hands, and then touched your eyes you have felt capsaicin in all of its awesome glory. Although, it probably did not feel awesome at that moment capsaicin is in fact very helpful in the relief of many illnesses including arthritis.

Arthritis, as I have discussed, is an inflammation of the joints. When joints get inflamed, something has to counter react the inflammation in order for relief from the pain. Cayenne peppers offer the ability to counter react the inflammation caused by arthritis. The capsaicin in cayenne pepper when used for anti-inflammatory purposes inhibits pain receptors in the nerves surrounding the infected joint from sending pain signals to the brain.

Modern medicine has cultivated the cayenne pepper into a number of creams for external use. These creams can be applied directly to the skin and offer effective anti-inflammatory qualities. Cayenne is also available as a supplement and can be taken orally. The supplement form of cayenne pepper is very effective in the treatment of arthritis symptoms, but it does take time to enter the body and work. Creams are the most popular form because of the fact that they offer a more instantaneous pain relief on contact.

Although the use of cayenne pepper for the treatment of arthritis is well tolerated by most people, there are some individuals who must be careful when using this form of relief. Cayenne pepper, as discussed, is very spicy. Individuals who are prone to heartburn could do more harm than good if cayenne is consumed. There is also the risk of gastrointestinal disorders and ulcers in certain individuals. Anyone who already had ulcers of the stomach or the intestines is strongly urged to stay away from cayenne pepper remedies of any kind as the spice can aggravate the ulcers. It is also suggested that anyone thinking of starting a cayenne pepper regime first consult their doctor and start slow with low doses of cayenne in order for your body to adjust to the peppers. There are some instances where individuals did not follow this instruction and took too much cayenne pepper, went into shock from the spice of the pepper. The shock did not last long, but is a wakeup call not to frighten your body with this surprisingly hot pepper.

It is also suggested that women who are pregnant avoid the use of cayenne peppers. Breastfeeding mothers also fall into this category. Children under two should never be given doses of cayenne pepper. If it can produce shock in a grown person, it can definitely have an effect on a person whose body is not fully developed. No one with an allergy to capsaicin should use cayenne pepper and it should never be applied to broken or irritated skin.

As has been stated previously, cayenne pepper can be used in a variety of over the counter remedies and supplements, but if the thought of chemically altered natural ingredients does not sit well with you, there are alternatives. Cayenne pepper can be added to all sorts of dishes to be naturally absorbed by the body, but there are also homemade remedies that may be used as well. These are applied directly to the skin and are surprisingly effective. Again, you are strongly cautioned in the use of these home remedies. Start slow and work up to where you feel comfortable. If any type of reaction occurs, stop the remedy immediately and seek medical attention if the reaction is severe. Here is a list of these remedies and how they can be made at home.

1. Castor oil and cayenne pepper can be mixed together. Soak a small towel in the mixture and apply it to sore joints. Start out with doing this for a few hours a day. If it works to relieve the pain in sore joint, try using it as overnight relief.

2. Buy cayenne pepper spice. This is the dried form of cayenne pepper and is available in any grocery store. Start out adding 1/8 of a teaspoon to your favorite recipes. A tablespoon per day of cayenne pepper is recommended for arthritis relief so slowly add more and work up to adding a tablespoon every day to your favorite foods. If you have children take caution in adding too much spice. The spice can be added to your individual plate after cooking.

3. Look for a brand of hot sauce that the main ingredient is "aged cayenne's." Apply the hot sauce a few times per day to any painful arthritis inflamed areas. This is effective in relieving arthritis pain. The only drawback reported with this remedy is the hot sauce has a tendency to stain clothes.

These three remedies can be effective in arthritis symptom relief and can help you avoid having to use many expensive pharmaceuticals.

In conclusion, there is no cure for arthritis. Any product claiming to be a cure is not to be trusted. People live longer these days and have many more responsibilities than in the past. Over time, the joints can give up. These joints can be replaced, but even with the advancements in modern medicines and the best doctors in the world, nothing is as good as the original joint. It is very important to take every step in the prevention of arthritis. The first and most important step is to make sure joints are lubricated properly. Drink plenty of water and get plenty of exercise every day. Movement is hard when the aches and pains of arthritis are a factor, but without movement, the body muscles and joints tend to seize up making movement all the more difficult. Try to walk more places than you drive. This can be better for your health and your wallet with the ever-growing gas prices.

Make a schedule for treatment. Write down your goals and how you want to treat your arthritis symptoms. Keep a diary of treatments that have worked, as well as treatments that may not have worked so well. Keep a list of questions for your doctor on hand, so you will not forget what you need to ask your doctor at your next check-up. Write down when symptoms occur. Keeping track of symptoms, over time, will give you a better indication of when a reaction might occur and what triggered the reaction. You will probably notice a pattern throughout the year. Flare-ups may occur at certain times of the year and not on others. The more you are aware of your arthritis the better treatment options can be employed to help with relief.

Finally, it is very important to educate the coming generation on arthritis and other ailments they may have to contend with later in life. The more our youth is educated in the areas of health, the less likely they are to make the same mistakes we made when we were younger. Over time, home remedies for certain ailments can be lost. People find it easier to get a prescription rather than ask grandma what she knows on the subject. Doctors are a wonderful source and a good one should be trusted, but with the economic decline we are facing these days, it is a good idea to educate the youth on inexpensive remedies that can be used rather than high priced chemically laced medicines. Communication is becoming a lost art in society. People hide behind phones and other devices so as not have to talk to other individuals. A good sense of community is a very effective tool in the treatment of arthritis. Your neighbor or friend may know of an arthritis remedy that could help that you have not heard of. We need to come together as a society in the prevention and treatment of medical conditions. Together, we can treat the symptoms we have today in hopes of one day finding a cure so the people of tomorrow will not know that arthritis was once "The Pain of the Century."

1. USEFUL ONLINE RESOURCES

www.mayoclinic.org

www.emedicinehealth.com

www.livestrong.com

www.arthritis-relief-natually.com

www.disabled-world.com

www.lifescript.com

www.livingstrong.com

www.webmd.com

www.all4naturalhealth.com

www.cayennepepper.info